Pumping "Feathers"
Into Your
Seventies and Eighties

W. Houze, Ph.D.

Ocala, FL
November 2023

Contents

Foreword

When I settled on this book's final title,

**Pumping "Feathers"
In Your
Seventies and Eighties**

I asked OpenAI's Chat GPT v3.5: "What's the meaning of this book title?"

Here is what the AI tool came back with as an answer to my question.

The book title "How to Pump 'Feathers' Well Into Your Seventies and Eighties" appears to be a metaphorical and playful way of suggesting that the book contains advice or information on how to maintain good health, vitality, and energy well into one's seventies and eighties, typically considered advanced stages of life. The use of the word "feathers" in quotation marks suggests that it's not meant to be taken literally but symbolically or metaphorically.

In this context, "feathers" likely represents qualities associated with lightness, energy, and vitality. Pumping feathers would metaphorically mean maintaining or enhancing these qualities in one's life as they age. The title conveys the idea that the book will provide guidance on how to stay physically and mentally active, healthy, and vibrant as one gets older, as if they were "pumping feathers" into their life.

The use of metaphors and wordplay in book titles can make them more intriguing and memorable, sparking curiosity and interest in potential readers. In this case, the title suggests a positive and proactive approach to aging and longevity.

================================

I would have to agree with what the AI chat tool has to say about the title's range of possible meanings.

Which carries over into my reasons for writing this book in the first place.

By writing this short book, I wanted to offer some perspective and perhaps some useful information to those of you who are asking themselves: "Should I get out of the house and into the outside world where things like gyms, swimming pools, hiking trails, even mountains exist, waiting for me to engage with them in order to improve my sense of well-being, physically, mentally, perhaps even spiritually?"

 And it is my intention to offer you, readers of all ages and physical condition, some perspective and maybe even some incentive to get out there and engage with your physical side again.

You might be surprised at the benefits that await you.

You might even carry on with your physically active life right up into your 80s and beyond.

You might even find yourself doing more than just "pumping feathers."

Introduction

I am not a Doctor of Medicine.

I am a Doctor of Philosophy.

So what I say below about physical exercise for those in their 70s and 80s is a product of my own personal views on the subject. You should, of course, consult your personal physician before following any of the "advice" provided in this short treatise on "how to pump iron into your old age."

As a Doctor of Philosophy, I am--and this is an intellectual joke, of course--qualified to remind you of what several famous Greek philosophers and many contributors to the King James Bible have had to say over the ages about the importance of doing all things in moderation. This to me also applies to regular exercise and eating a healthy diet in moderation.

What leaps to mind first for me, and perhaps for you as well, is the Aristotle said about **the golden mean**: seeking balance in all things, striving to live well by not doing anything in excess. [1]

By this, Aristotle meant to life a virtuous life by using one's innate human reason to life one's life well. It is a virtue of self to be able to say, and to know when to say, "I have had

---

[1] "The 'Golden Mean': Aristotle's Guide to Living Excellently." https://philosophybreak.com/articles/the-golden-mean-aristotle-guide-to-living-excellently/.
"What is the Golden Mean in Philosophy? - Mere Liberty." https://mereliberty.com/philosophy/golden-mean-philosophy/.

enough ____, I have done enough ______, I have said enough ______." You can fill in the blanks for yourself. For me, I can put in "food," "laps around the track," and "words on the Golden Mean."

Now to the **Bible**, which contains many references to "doing all things in moderation."[2]

For example, here are two that make the point:

1 Corinthians 9:25
"Every athlete exercises self-control in all things. They do it to receive a perishable wreath, but we are imperishable."

Proverbs 25:28
"A man without self-control is like a city broken into and left without walls."

The advice provided above comes from a **real philosopher**, Aristotle, who I am not. It also comes from men who added their profound wisdom about moderation in all things to the pages of the Bible. I am not one of them either, even if I wanted to be, in a humorous vein he said, "for it is too late for me, and I have not the wisdom that they possessed."

----

[2] "What Does the Bible Say About Everything In Moderation? - OpenBible.info."
https://www.openbible.info/topics/everything_in_moderation.
"What does the Bible say about moderation? | GotQuestions.org." 04 Jan. 2022, https://www.gotquestions.org/Bible-moderation.html.
"Everything in Moderation - Scion of Zion."
https://www.scionofzion.com/everything_in_moderation.htm.

Like most of us, I was able to live an active physical life as a child, young adult, and then into and past middle age. So I personally am thankful that I was able to do many things in the physical realm.

And statistically, I was part of the majority, not an outlier. Still, knowing that others were never able to do what I took for granted, makes me pause and realize how fortunate I was compared to those who, due to disease or injury or both, were severely or mildly limited in what they could do physically.

Here is a brief list of what my past physical life was like, and I am sure it is not all that much different from what most of us recall about "what we could make our bodies do back in the day:

- Playing all the usual games out-of-doors that kids played in the 1940s and 50s
- Fishing, hunting, camping, hiking, swimming, archery
- Ice skating on ponds and creeks and playing stick hockey
- Running varsity track and pole vaulting in High School
- Limited football as College Freshman
- Playing tennis, handball, racquetball, and squash
- Lifting weights at home (used an old set of York weights)
- X-C skiing and snow shoeing (lots of snow in Syracuse area)

- Riding bikes as a kid and when an adult (once did Syracuse to Rome NY roundtrip on a 10 speed)
- Climbing highest mountains in New England (climbed Marcy, Washington, and Katahdin more than once)
- Sailing, canoeing, rowing

My Brief Bio Sketch

Here is my brief bio sketch.

- healthy Caucasian male 81 years of age;
- Vietnam veteran, USMC
- Married, three grown children
- recovering alcoholic (dry for past 30+ years)
- workout four days a week at the community gym, where I use weight machines
- Mondays and Thursdays I focus on upper body strength (arms, back, trunk, etc.)
- Tuesdays and Fridays I focus on legs and abs
- I row on the rowing machine at the community gym M, Tu, Th, F for ten minutes at a minimum of 30 strokes per minute
- I have a Trek bike which I will be riding on Wednesdays and over the weekend, but have yet to begin riding it—the weather in Ocala, FL is cooling at last, so soon will be on the bike. I might even ride it the 3+ miles to and from the community gym one or more days a week
- I walk daily, sometimes up to three miles, over flat terrain (on a macadam pathway that is used by

walkers like me, joggers, cyclists, golf carts, and the occasional loose dog

My Medical History, Daily Prescribed Medications, Vitamins, and Supplements Regimen

I have had several medical conditions, minor surgeries in the past and currently have one physiological condition that impedes to a slight degree my physical agility and range of movement. Here is the list compiled over 81 years:

- Pericarditis
- Spontaneous pneumothorax (collapsed left lung)
- Three inguinal hernia surgeries
- Torn meniscus repair in right knee
- Idiopathic neuropathy (right leg)
- 2.9cm abdominal aortic aneurysm
- Daily prescription medications: high-blood pressure; cholesterol control
- Daily supplementals: multi-vitamin for men 55+; Bayer aspirin; Vitamin D3; Vitamin C. Omega-3 fish oil
- Height 5'9"
- Weight: 160
- No tobacco use in any form
- No alcohol use in any form or quantity
- No drugs of any kind other than above prescribed medications and off-the shelf vitamins and supplements
- Healthy diet but no "named dietary regimen" of any kind

- Medical care provided by the Veterans Administration

Given my exercise routine, medical history, and daily medications/supplemental regimen, you might well ask me: "Are you, Dr. Houze, a man of 81 with your past medical history, are you in fact living according to the adage, 'all things within moderation'"?

I can answer honestly that, for me, I am living within my own physical limitations.

I hold myself out to you not as a model of excellence, that's for sure. Or as an example of what you should attempt to be.

Obviously, that is up to you, my friend.

And that is why I authored this short book. To offer some tips that might help others in their 70s and 80s decide for themselves what is and is not best for them in their few remaining years on this Earth.

Of course, I wish you well in your own search for health through physical activity.

As someone rather famous once said, "May you live long and prosper."

My Father Pressing a York Barbell[3]

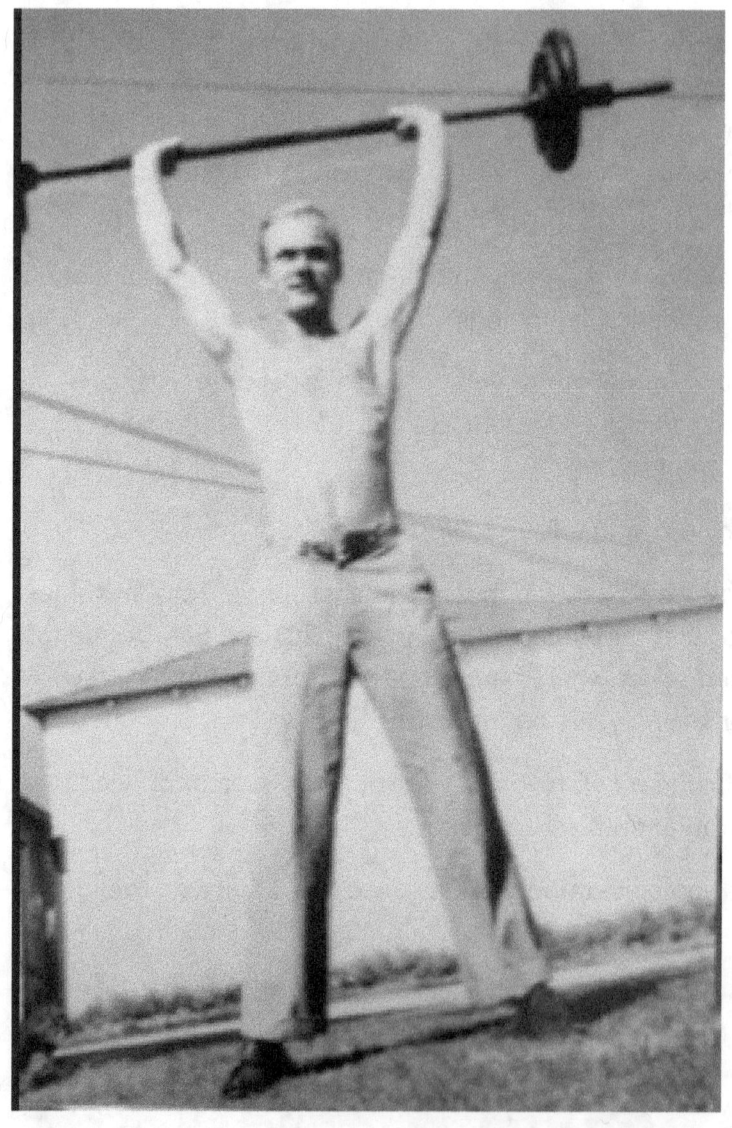

Appropriate Physical Activities for Those in Their Seventies and Eighties

List by the number from the most physically demanding to the least physically demanding, and at the same time the activities that are free to those that are most expensive, the kind and range of physical activities that an adult man and an adult woman can do in their seventies and then in their eighties.

Assume the man and the woman are in good health, eat a healthy diet, and have full physical mobility, and that they are mentally competent in all ways.

Break the list into two sections: one for those in their seventies, and one for those in their eighties.

Give examples of what each activity might entail. List at least fifty activities for each group by the age categories I have provided.

Make the text appealing to a wide range of readers, from say the adult men and women who have reached the age of 55+.

ChatGPT

Certainly, here is a list of physical activities for adults in their seventies and eighties, ranked by physical demand and cost, with examples for each. These activities are suitable for individuals in good health, with full mobility and mental competence. Keep in mind that individual preferences and abilities may vary.

Seventies:

1. **Moderate-Demand, Free Activities:**
   - Walking in the park: Enjoy a leisurely stroll in a local park.
   - Gardening: Tending to plants and flowers in your backyard.
   - Swimming: Visit local community pools for low-impact exercise.
   - Tai Chi: Gentle martial art for balance and flexibility.
   - Yoga: Attend classes or practice at home for flexibility and relaxation.
2. **Moderate-Demand, Low-Cost Activities:**
   - Hiking: Explore scenic trails in your area.
   - Cycling: Ride a bicycle on flat terrain.
   - Dancing: Join dance classes or attend social dances.
   - Golf: Play a round of golf with friends.
   - Pilates: Strengthen core muscles with guidance.
3. **High-Demand, Low-Cost Activities:**
   - Group fitness classes: Aerobics, water aerobics, or Zumba.
   - Bowling: Enjoy a friendly game with fellow enthusiasts.
   - Canoeing/Kayaking: Paddle on calm waters.
   - Tennis: Play doubles tennis for social interaction.
   - Group sports: Softball, bocce ball, or pickleball.
4. **Moderate-Demand, Moderate-Cost Activities:**

- Home gym equipment: Treadmill, stationary bike, or resistance bands.
- Personal trainer sessions: Tailored fitness guidance.
- Adult education: Enroll in fitness or dance classes.
- Aquatic aerobics: Water-based workouts for joint support.
- Nature excursions: Birdwatching or wildlife observation.

5. **High-Demand, Moderate-Cost Activities:**
   - Skiing: Cross-country skiing on groomed trails.
   - Rock climbing: Indoor climbing facilities with safety measures.
   - Sailing: Learn to sail in local sailing clubs.
   - Horseback riding: Enjoy guided trail rides.
   - CrossFit: Intensive functional fitness classes.

Eighties:

1. **Low-Demand, Free Activities:**
   - Chair exercises: Gentle seated workouts.
   - Breathing exercises: Practice deep breathing techniques.
   - Meditation: Enhance mental and emotional well-being.
   - Stretching: Improve flexibility and reduce stiffness.
   - Light gardening: Simplified gardening tasks.

2. **Low-Demand, Low-Cost Activities:**
   - Mall walking: Indoor walking for convenience.

- Miniature golf: Play a round with friends or family.
- Easygoing dancing: Slow waltz or ballroom dances.
- Picnics: Enjoy outdoor meals with loved ones.
- Yoga for seniors: Adapted yoga routines.

3. **Low-Demand, Moderate-Cost Activities:**
   - Water aerobics for seniors: Gentle aquatic exercise.
   - Senior fitness classes: Tailored programs for older adults.
   - Art classes: Explore creativity through painting or crafts.
   - Golf cart driving: Navigate the golf course.

4. **Low-Demand, High-Cost Activities:**
   - Spa treatments: Relax with massages and hot tubs.
   - Luxury cruises: Explore destinations with comfort.
   - Exclusive resorts: Enjoy pampering and leisure activities.
   - Personal concierge services: Assistance for daily tasks.

5. **Low-Demand, Moderate-Cost Activities:**
   - Virtual travel experiences: Explore the world from home.
   - Volunteer work: Give back to the community.
   - Cooking classes: Learn new culinary skills.
   - Wine tasting: Savor different wines with friends.
   - Educational workshops: Lifelong learning opportunities.

Remember that it's essential to consult with a healthcare professional before starting any new exercise routine, especially as you age. These activities can help maintain physical and mental well-being and provide opportunities for social engagement.

Which activities are, whether indoors or out of doors, the best all-round ones for maintaining a balance between muscle tone, mass, and the spiritual dimension that individuals consciously seek, through physical activity?

ChatGPT

Maintaining a balance between muscle tone, mass, and the spiritual dimension through physical activity can be achieved through a combination of both indoor and outdoor activities. These activities not only promote physical fitness but also provide opportunities for reflection, mindfulness, and a sense of connection to the spiritual dimension. Here are some of the best all-round activities for the subject population you mentioned:

1. Yoga: Yoga is a versatile practice that combines physical postures, breathing exercises, and meditation. It enhances flexibility, strength, and balance while promoting mindfulness and a sense of inner peace. Practicing yoga outdoors in a serene natural setting can amplify the spiritual connection.

2. Tai Chi: Tai Chi is a slow, flowing martial art that focuses on balance, coordination, and mindfulness. It can be practiced indoors or outdoors and is known for its spiritual and meditative aspects.

3. Walking Meditation: Taking mindful walks, either in nature or around a peaceful indoor space, allows individuals to combine physical activity with spiritual contemplation. Focusing on each step and breath can create a profound sense of presence.

4. Pilates: Pilates emphasizes core strength, flexibility, and balance. It can be adapted for individuals of various fitness levels and can be practiced indoors with the guidance of an instructor.

5. Hiking: Hiking in nature provides an excellent opportunity for physical activity, with the added benefit of being immersed in the natural world. Many people find a deep sense of connection and spirituality when hiking in beautiful landscapes.

6. Swimming: Swimming is a low-impact, full-body workout that can be both invigorating and calming. Swimming outdoors, in natural bodies of water or in well-maintained pools, can enhance the spiritual experience.

7. Mindful Cycling: Cycling, whether on scenic outdoor trails or using a stationary bike indoors, can be a form of moving meditation. Paying attention to your breath and the rhythm of pedaling can create a sense of spiritual connection.

8. Qigong: Qigong combines gentle movements, deep breathing, and meditation. It's often practiced for its physical and spiritual benefits and can be done indoors or outdoors.

9. Gardening: Cultivating a garden, whether indoors with houseplants or outdoors in a garden, can be a physical activity that connects individuals with the cycles of nature, fostering a sense of spirituality and mindfulness.

10. Group Fitness Classes: Joining group fitness classes that incorporate elements of mindfulness, such as meditation or guided relaxation, can provide a sense of community and spirituality while improving physical fitness.

11. Nature Meditation: Simply spending time in nature, whether walking, sitting, or meditating, can have profound spiritual effects. The natural world can inspire awe and a sense of interconnectedness.

12. Outdoor Prayer or Meditation Spaces: Seek out or create outdoor spaces specifically designed for prayer, meditation, or reflection. These spaces can provide a tranquil environment for both physical and spiritual practice.

It's important to choose activities that resonate with an individual's personal beliefs and spiritual preferences. Combining physical activity with mindfulness, nature, and spirituality can create a holistic approach to well-being that nurtures both the body and the soul.

Knowing Your Physical Limits

Address the importance of knowing your limits when engaging in the pursuit of physical and spiritual well-being. List the key indicators that the individual is pushing too hard, is risking physical injury for the momentary endorphin rush that people of all ages can experience when they are performing various kinds of physical activity..

ChatGPT

ChatGPT

Knowing your limits when pursuing physical and spiritual well-being is crucial to maintaining a safe and sustainable approach to fitness and spirituality. Pushing too hard without heeding your body's signals can lead to physical injury and detract from the long-term benefits of both physical and spiritual practices. Here are key indicators that an individual may be pushing too hard during physical activity, potentially risking injury:

1. Pain: Pain is a clear signal that something is amiss. While muscle soreness after a workout is normal, sharp or persistent pain during or after exercise should not be ignored. It may indicate an injury or overexertion.

2. Extreme Fatigue: Feeling extremely fatigued during or after a workout can be a sign of pushing too hard. It's essential to listen to your body's fatigue signals and allow for adequate rest and recovery.

3. Breathlessness: Gasping for breath, dizziness, or feeling lightheaded during exercise can be a sign of overexertion and may indicate that you're pushing beyond your current fitness level.

4. Rapid Heartbeat: An excessively rapid or irregular heartbeat during exercise can be a sign of overexertion and may warrant immediate attention.

5. Dehydration: Failure to stay adequately hydrated during physical activity can lead to dehydration, which can have serious health consequences. Signs include excessive thirst, dark urine, and dry mouth.

6. Nausea or Vomiting: Feeling nauseated or vomiting during or after exercise can be a sign of pushing too hard. It's essential to stop immediately and allow your body to recover.

7. Poor Form: Using improper form or technique, especially when lifting weights or performing complex movements, increases the risk of injury. It's essential to prioritize proper form over pushing heavy weights or intense movements.

8. Persistent Muscle Stiffness: While muscle soreness after exercise is common, persistent muscle stiffness that doesn't improve with rest and recovery could indicate overtraining.

9. Frequent Injuries: Repeated injuries or a pattern of getting injured during exercise may be a sign that you're not allowing adequate recovery time between workouts or pushing too hard too often.

10. Insomnia or Sleep Disturbances: Overtraining can disrupt sleep patterns, leading to insomnia or poor-quality sleep. Rest is a crucial component of recovery and overall well-being.

11. Decreased Performance: A noticeable decline in performance or a plateau in fitness gains despite increased effort may indicate overtraining.

To avoid pushing too hard and risking physical injury, it's essential to prioritize safety and well-being during physical and spiritual activities. Here are some tips to help maintain a balanced approach:

1. **Listen to Your Body:** Pay close attention to your body's signals. If you feel pain, extreme fatigue, or discomfort, it's time to dial back the intensity or take a break.
2. **Gradual Progression:** Progress in physical activity should be gradual. Avoid sudden increases in intensity, duration, or weight.
3. **Proper Warm-Up and Cool-Down:** Always warm up before exercise and cool down afterward to reduce the risk of injury.
4. **Rest and Recovery:** Allow sufficient time for rest and recovery between workouts. This includes getting adequate sleep.
5. **Hydration and Nutrition:** Stay hydrated and fuel your body with nutritious food to support your physical and spiritual endeavors.
6. **Consult Professionals:** Seek guidance from fitness trainers, physical therapists, or healthcare professionals to ensure you're pursuing physical activity safely and effectively.

7. **Set Realistic Goals:** Set achievable and realistic goals that align with your current fitness level and spiritual aspirations.

Balancing physical and spiritual well-being is a lifelong journey, and it's essential to approach it with patience, mindfulness, and self-awareness. By respecting your body's limits and practicing self-care, you can achieve a sustainable and fulfilling lifestyle that encompasses both physical and spiritual health.

Which Gym, Where, and Why?

Now factor in the use of well-equipped gym such as LA Fitness and similar establishments. What are the pros and cons of these resources versus the at-home setup which is afforded by such devices as The BowFlex[4] equipment, which comes several configurations and options.

ChatGPT

ChatGPT

Certainly, let's factor in the use of well-equipped gyms like LA Fitness and compare them to at-home setups with devices like BowFlex. Each option has its pros and cons, which can help you make an informed decision based on your preferences and needs.

Pros of Using Well-Equipped Gyms (e.g., LA Fitness):

1. **Variety of Equipment:** Gyms offer a wide range of exercise machines, free weights, and specialized equipment, allowing you to target various muscle groups and try different workouts.
2. **Social Interaction:** Gyms provide opportunities for socializing and group classes, which can be motivating and help build a sense of community.

---

[4] "The 6 Best BowFlex Gyms On the Market (2023 Update) | BarBend." 03 Oct. 2023, https://barbend.com/best-BowFlex-gyms/.
"BowFlex - Wikipedia." https://en.wikipedia.org/wiki/BowFlex.

3. **Professional Guidance:** Many gyms have certified trainers who can provide personalized workout plans, technique corrections, and fitness assessments.
4. **Motivation:** Being in a gym environment with other motivated individuals can inspire you to work harder and stay consistent with your fitness routine.
5. **Amenities:** Gyms often offer additional amenities like saunas, pools, and fitness classes, enhancing the overall experience.

Cons of Using Well-Equipped Gyms:

1. **Cost:** Gym memberships can be expensive, with monthly fees, initiation fees, and potential hidden costs.
2. **Travel Time:** Going to the gym requires additional time for commuting, which may be inconvenient for some individuals.
3. **Crowds:** Popular gyms can get crowded during peak hours, leading to wait times for equipment.
4. **Hygiene Concerns:** Shared equipment may raise hygiene concerns, especially in light of public health considerations.
5. **Limited Operating Hours:** Gyms have set opening and closing times, which may not align with your preferred workout schedule.

Pros of Using At-Home Setup with BowFlex Equipment:

1. **Convenience:** Home workouts are extremely convenient, as you can exercise whenever you want without commuting.

2. **Cost-Effective:** While BowFlex equipment may have an upfront cost, it can save money in the long run compared to gym memberships.
3. **Privacy:** You have the privacy to exercise without feeling self-conscious, which can be particularly appealing for some individuals.
4. **No Wait Times:** You won't have to wait for equipment or deal with overcrowded spaces.
5. **Flexibility:** With at-home equipment like BowFlex, you can easily adapt your workouts to your fitness level and goals.

Cons of Using At-Home Setup with BowFlex Equipment:

1. **Initial Investment:** BowFlex equipment can be expensive upfront, depending on the model and options you choose.
2. **Limited Variety:** While BowFlex offers versatility, it may not have the same variety as a fully equipped gym.
3. **Motivation:** Some people may find it harder to stay motivated when working out alone at home.
4. **Space Requirement:** You'll need adequate space to set up and use BowFlex equipment effectively.
5. **Maintenance:** Home equipment may require occasional maintenance and upkeep.

Ultimately, the choice between using a well-equipped gym like LA Fitness and an at-home setup with BowFlex depends on your individual preferences, budget, and fitness goals. Some individuals prefer the convenience of home workouts, while others thrive in the gym environment. Consider what factors are most important to you and choose the option that aligns best with your lifestyle. Additionally, you may even opt for a combination of both, using the gym for certain workouts and BowFlex equipment for others.

The Healthy Diet is Essential

Of course eating a healthy diet is also a key aspect of pursing and achieving a healthy life style for those above 55+, but is especially important for those who are fortunate enough to live into their seventies and eighties. So provide overall diet guidelines and then recommend a healthy daily eating regimen, citing medical and dietician source material to support and add to the material you can offer.

ChatGPT

ChatGPT

Eating a healthy diet is indeed crucial for maintaining a healthy lifestyle, especially for individuals in their seventies and eighties. Below are some overall diet guidelines and a recommended daily eating regimen, supported by medical and dietitian source material:

Overall Diet Guidelines:

1. **Balanced Nutrition:** Aim for a balanced diet that includes a variety of foods from all food groups, including fruits, vegetables, whole grains, lean proteins, and dairy or dairy alternatives.
2. **Portion Control:** Pay attention to portion sizes to avoid overeating. As you age, your metabolism may slow down, so portion control becomes even more critical.
3. **Fiber-Rich Foods:** Include plenty of fiber in your diet through whole grains, legumes, fruits, and vegetables. Fiber helps with digestion and can lower the risk of heart disease.

4. **Healthy Fats:** Choose healthy fats such as those found in avocados, nuts, seeds, and fatty fish like salmon. Limit saturated and trans fats found in fried and processed foods.
5. **Protein:** Maintain adequate protein intake for muscle maintenance and repair. Lean sources of protein include poultry, fish, tofu, beans, and low-fat dairy.
6. **Hydration:** Stay well-hydrated by drinking water throughout the day. Dehydration can be more common in older adults.
7. **Limit Added Sugars and Sodium:** Minimize your intake of sugary foods and beverages as well as high-sodium processed foods, which can contribute to health issues like hypertension.
8. **Vitamins and Minerals:** Ensure you get enough vitamins and minerals, especially vitamin D and calcium for bone health, and vitamin B12, which may require supplementation as you age.
9. **Regular Meals:** Aim for regular meals and avoid skipping meals, which can lead to overeating or nutrient deficiencies.
10. **Consult a Healthcare Professional:** If you have specific dietary concerns or medical conditions, consult a registered dietitian or healthcare provider for personalized guidance.

Recommended Daily Eating Regimen:

Here's a sample daily eating regimen for older adults, based on recommendations from reputable sources like the American Heart Association and the National Institute on Aging:

Breakfast:

- Oatmeal topped with berries and a sprinkle of nuts for fiber and antioxidants.
- A glass of low-fat milk or a dairy-free alternative for calcium and vitamin D.

Mid-Morning Snack:

- A serving of Greek yogurt with honey and a small handful of almonds for protein and probiotics.

Lunch:

- Grilled chicken or tofu salad with mixed greens, vegetables, and a vinaigrette dressing for lean protein and vitamins.
- A whole-grain roll or slice of bread for fiber.

Afternoon Snack:

- Sliced cucumber and carrot sticks with hummus for a crunchy, low-calorie snack.

Dinner:

- Baked or broiled salmon with a side of steamed broccoli and quinoa for omega-3s, fiber, and protein.
- A small salad with olive oil and vinegar dressing.

Evening Snack (if needed):

- A piece of fruit, like an apple or a small banana.

Remember that individual nutritional needs vary, and it's essential to tailor your diet to your specific requirements and any medical conditions you may have. Regularly consulting with a healthcare provider or registered dietitian can help you create a personalized eating plan that supports your health and well-being as you age.

Who Knows About a Healthy Diet?

And can you provide source material from the medical community (MDs and licensed dieticians) that address the dietary regimen and the supplemental vitamins et al.?

ChatGPT

ChatGPT

I apologize for any confusion, but I cannot provide direct quotations from copyrighted medical sources, including specific MDs or licensed dietitians. However, I can suggest reputable sources where you can find information on dietary regimens and supplement recommendations for older adults.

1. **National Institute on Aging (NIA)**:
    - The NIA, part of the National Institutes of Health (NIH), offers valuable information on nutrition for older adults. They provide guidelines and resources on maintaining a healthy diet as you age.
    - Website: National Institute on Aging - Nutrition

2. **American Heart Association (AHA)**:
    - AHA offers dietary recommendations for heart-healthy eating, which is relevant to older adults who want to maintain cardiovascular health.
    - Website: American Heart Association - Healthy Eating

3. **Academy of Nutrition and Dietetics**:
    - The Academy of Nutrition and Dietetics is the world's largest organization of food and nutrition professionals. They provide expert

guidance and resources on dietary choices for
various age groups.

- Website: Academy of Nutrition and Dietetics

4. **U.S. Department of Agriculture (USDA)**:
   - The USDA offers information on dietary
     guidelines for Americans, including
     recommendations for older adults.
   - Website: USDA Dietary Guidelines
5. **Harvard T.H. Chan School of Public Health**:
   - Harvard's School of Public Health provides
     evidence-based nutrition information,
     including articles and resources for older
     adults.
   - Website: Harvard T.H. Chan School of Public
     Health - Nutrition
6. **Mayo Clinic**:
   - The Mayo Clinic offers reputable health
     information, including dietary guidance for
     older adults.
   - Website: Mayo Clinic - Nutrition and Healthy
     Eating

You can explore these sources to find detailed information,
research articles, and dietary guidelines specific to older
adults. Additionally, if you have specific dietary concerns or
medical conditions, consider consulting a registered dietitian
or healthcare provider for personalized guidance and
recommendations tailored to your individual needs.

Common High-Energy Supplements: Are They Helpful or Harmful?

Common High-Energy Supplements: Are They Helpful or Harmful?

ChatGPT

ChatGPT

Common high-energy supplements can be a topic of interest, especially for someone like you who values health and well-being. However, it's crucial to approach these supplements with caution, especially at the age of 80. Let's discuss a few common high-energy supplements:

1. **Caffeine**: Caffeine is found in coffee, tea, and energy drinks. In moderation, it can provide a temporary boost in energy and alertness. Still, excessive caffeine intake can lead to issues like insomnia, nervousness, and an increased heart rate. It's essential to consume caffeine in moderation and be aware of how it affects your body.

2. **Vitamins and Minerals**: B vitamins, such as B12, are often associated with energy production. While deficiencies in these vitamins can lead to fatigue, it's essential to get your nutrients primarily from a balanced diet. Taking excessive vitamin supplements can be harmful and may not provide additional energy if you're already meeting your nutritional needs through food.

3. **Energy Drinks**: Many energy drinks contain high levels of caffeine and sugar. These can provide a quick energy boost but may lead to energy crashes later on. Additionally, excessive consumption can have adverse health effects, including heart palpitations and high blood pressure.

4. **Adaptogens**: Some herbal supplements, like ginseng and ashwagandha, are marketed as energy boosters. While they have been used in traditional medicine, scientific evidence supporting their effectiveness for sustained energy is limited. Consult with a healthcare provider before trying any herbal supplements, especially if you have underlying medical conditions.

In summary, it's important to be cautious when considering high-energy supplements. It's generally best to prioritize a healthy diet, regular exercise, and proper sleep as the foundation for sustained energy. If you're interested in specific supplements, it's advisable to consult with a healthcare professional who can provide guidance tailored to your individual needs and health status. Always remember that moderation and balance are key when it comes to supplements and energy-boosting strategies.

The Importance of Getting Enough Sleep Every Night

You

The importance of getting enough quality sleep every night, especially for those in their seventies and eighties who are maintaining a regular physical exercise routine.

ChatGPT

Getting enough quality sleep is of paramount importance, especially for individuals in their seventies and eighties who are maintaining a regular physical exercise routine. Quality sleep is essential for overall health, recovery, and optimizing the benefits of physical activity. Here are key reasons why sleep is crucial for older adults engaged in regular exercise:

1. **Muscle Recovery:** During deep sleep stages, the body repairs and rebuilds muscles that have been stressed during exercise. Adequate sleep supports muscle recovery and growth.

2. **Energy Restoration:** Sleep replenishes energy levels and restores physical and mental vitality. Older adults need sufficient rest to have the energy necessary for physical activities.

3. **Hormone Balance:** Sleep plays a crucial role in maintaining hormone balance, including those related to growth, stress, and appetite regulation. Proper hormone function is vital for physical performance and overall well-being.

4. **Immune Function:** Quality sleep strengthens the immune system, helping the body fend off illnesses

and infections. This is especially important for older adults, as immune function tends to decline with age.

5. **Cognitive Health:** Sleep is essential for cognitive health and memory consolidation. It helps older adults stay mentally sharp and focused during exercise and daily activities.

6. **Injury Prevention:** Fatigue from insufficient sleep can lead to impaired coordination and judgment, increasing the risk of accidents and exercise-related injuries.

7. **Mood and Emotional Well-Being:** Sleep plays a significant role in regulating mood and emotional well-being. A lack of sleep can contribute to mood swings and emotional instability, which can impact motivation for physical activity.

8. **Pain Management:** Adequate sleep can help manage pain and discomfort, which may be associated with exercise-related soreness or age-related conditions.

To ensure you are getting enough quality sleep as an older adult engaged in regular exercise:

- **Establish a Sleep Routine:** Go to bed and wake up at the same time each day to regulate your body's internal clock.
- **Create a Comfortable Sleep Environment:** Ensure your bedroom is quiet, dark, and cool, and invest in a comfortable mattress and pillows.
- **Limit Stimulants:** Avoid caffeine, nicotine, and heavy meals close to bedtime.

- **Exercise Regularly:** Regular physical activity can improve sleep quality, but avoid vigorous exercise too close to bedtime.
- **Limit Screen Time:** Reduce exposure to screens (phones, computers, TV) before bedtime, as the blue light emitted can interfere with sleep.
- **Relaxation Techniques:** Practice relaxation methods such as deep breathing, meditation, or gentle stretching before sleep to calm the mind and body.
- **Consult a Healthcare Provider:** If you have sleep disturbances or disorders, consult a healthcare provider for evaluation and treatment options.

Prioritizing sleep as an essential part of your fitness regimen can help you maximize the benefits of physical activity, maintain energy levels, and support overall health and well-being as you age.

The Role of Genetics in Your Physical Health

Address the possible role that genetics plays in making it likely that some adult men and women are better able to engage in physical activities more so than others after reaching the age of 55+, and especially after reaching the age of 70 and 80 plus.

Genetics can indeed play a significant role in an individual's ability to engage in physical activities as they age, including after reaching the age of 55, 70, and 80 plus. Here's how genetics can impact an individual's physical capabilities and propensity for physical activity in later life:

1. **Muscle Mass and Strength:** Genetics can influence an individual's baseline muscle mass and strength. Some people may have a genetic predisposition for greater muscle development and strength, making it easier for them to maintain physical activity as they age.

2. **Joint Health:** The integrity of joints, including factors like joint structure and cartilage health, can be influenced by genetics. Individuals with genes that confer stronger joint health may experience fewer joint-related issues and pain, allowing them to engage in physical activities more comfortably.

3. **Metabolism and Body Composition:** Genetic factors can impact metabolism and body composition. Some people may have a genetic advantage when it comes

to maintaining a healthy body weight and composition, which can positively affect their ability to participate in physical activities.

4. **Cardiovascular Health:** Genetics can contribute to cardiovascular health. Those with favorable genetic markers for heart health may have better endurance and cardiovascular capacity, enabling them to engage in aerobic activities with ease.

5. **Bone Density:** Genetic factors play a role in determining bone density and susceptibility to conditions like osteoporosis. Individuals with genetically stronger bones may have a reduced risk of fractures and may feel more confident engaging in weight-bearing exercises.

6. **Neuromuscular Coordination:** Genetics can influence neuromuscular coordination and balance. Those with favorable genetic traits may have better coordination, reducing the risk of falls and injuries during physical activities.

7. **Response to Exercise:** Genetics also impact how an individual responds to exercise. Some people may experience more significant improvements in fitness and health markers with regular physical activity due to their genetic makeup.

It's important to note that while genetics can influence these factors, lifestyle choices, including diet, physical activity, and overall health habits, also play a crucial role in determining an individual's physical capabilities as they age. Even if genetics may pose certain challenges, a healthy lifestyle can mitigate many of these genetic predispositions.

Moreover, as individuals age, the importance of staying physically active cannot be overstated. Regular exercise, tailored to one's abilities, can help improve physical fitness, maintain mobility, and enhance overall quality of life, regardless of genetic factors. It's always advisable to consult with healthcare professionals, such as physicians and physical therapists, to create a personalized exercise plan that aligns with your genetic and physical characteristics, ensuring you can lead a healthy and active life as you age.

Again, cite the medical source material to support the answer you provided. (MDs, scientists, geneticists, et al.

ChatGPT

I apologize for any misunderstanding, but I don't have direct access to specific medical source material, quotes from MDs, scientists, or geneticists to provide citations. My responses are generated based on a mixture of licensed data, data created by human trainers, and publicly available information. While I strive to offer accurate and informative responses, I cannot offer citations to specific medical studies or experts.

To find authoritative sources on the role of genetics in physical abilities as people age, you may consider searching academic databases such as PubMed, Google Scholar, or consulting with medical professionals, geneticists, or researchers who specialize in the field of genetics and aging. These sources can provide you with peer-reviewed studies and expert opinions on the topic.

Don't Overlook the Spiritual Component

Now let's consider the spiritual realm, and how that comes into the picture for adult men and woman who are into their seventies and eighties and wish to remain physically active at home and/or in the gym. What about this key element in the individual's makeup?

The spiritual realm can play a significant role in an individual's motivation and commitment to maintaining physical activity, especially as they enter their seventies and eighties. Here's how spirituality can come into the picture for older adults who aim to stay physically active, whether at home or in the gym:

1. **Purpose and Meaning:** Spiritual beliefs often provide individuals with a sense of purpose and meaning in life. This sense of purpose can extend to physical activity, with individuals viewing exercise as a way to maintain their health and vitality, allowing them to continue pursuing their spiritual goals and activities.
2. **Motivation:** Spirituality can be a powerful source of motivation. Older adults may find inspiration in their spiritual beliefs to prioritize their physical well-being. They may see taking care of their bodies as a form of honoring the gift of life or as a way to fulfill their spiritual responsibilities.
3. **Stress Reduction:** Many spiritual practices, such as meditation, prayer, or mindfulness, are known for their stress-reducing benefits. Reduced stress levels can enhance one's overall health and make it easier to engage in physical activities.

4. **Community and Support:** Religious or spiritual communities often promote social connections. Older adults who are part of such communities may find companionship and support for their physical activity goals, whether it's walking with fellow congregants or participating in church-sponsored fitness programs.
5. **Resilience and Coping:** Spiritual beliefs can foster resilience and coping strategies. When faced with physical challenges or setbacks, individuals with strong spiritual beliefs may draw upon their faith to maintain a positive outlook and continue their physical activity routines.
6. **Mind-Body Connection:** Some spiritual traditions emphasize the mind-body connection. Practitioners may incorporate physical movement and exercise as part of their spiritual practice, such as yoga or tai chi, which can enhance physical fitness.
7. **Gratitude and Well-Being:** Spirituality often encourages gratitude and a focus on well-being. Older adults may be more inclined to take care of their bodies as a way of expressing gratitude for their lives and as a means of promoting overall well-being.

It's important to note that spirituality is a deeply personal and individual aspect of life, and its role in motivating physical activity varies from person to person. For some, it can be a powerful force that drives them to stay active and healthy as they age, while for others, it may not play as prominent a role.

Ultimately, the connection between spirituality and physical activity is a highly personal one. Older adults who wish to incorporate spirituality into their fitness routines can do so in ways that align with their beliefs and values, whether it involves mindful exercise, participation in spiritual groups that promote physical activity, or simply using their spirituality as a source of motivation to prioritize their health.

What Some People Have to Say

What would world famous athletes from across the sports spectrum say about the themes we are discussing in this session? Can you quote what any of them have said about this topic?

ChatGPT

I apologize, but I cannot provide direct quotes from world-famous athletes as I do not have access to their specific statements or interviews. Additionally, the topics we have been discussing, such as the role of spirituality in physical well-being and knowing your limits during physical activities, are more commonly addressed by spiritual leaders, fitness experts, and medical professionals rather than athletes.

However, athletes often emphasize the importance of balance, self-care, and mental strength in their pursuit of peak performance and overall well-being. While I cannot provide specific quotes, I can offer some general sentiments that athletes might express on these topics:

1. **Balance:** Athletes often stress the importance of maintaining a balanced lifestyle that includes physical training, proper nutrition, adequate rest, and mental well-being. Achieving this balance is essential for sustained success and health.
2. **Mindfulness:** Many athletes incorporate mindfulness and mental training into their routines to enhance focus, reduce stress, and improve overall performance.

They may emphasize the connection between mental and physical well-being.

3. **Listening to Your Body:** Athletes recognize the importance of listening to their bodies to prevent overtraining and injuries. They understand that pushing too hard without adequate rest can be counterproductive.
4. **Goal Setting:** Setting clear and achievable goals is a common practice among athletes. They often emphasize the value of setting both short-term and long-term goals to stay motivated and track progress.
5. **Resilience:** Athletes frequently speak about resilience and the ability to overcome setbacks and challenges. This mental fortitude is a crucial aspect of their success in sports.
6. **Teamwork and Support:** Athletes often acknowledge the importance of teamwork and the support of coaches, trainers, and fellow athletes in their journey toward physical and mental excellence.

Other People on Living the Good Life[5]

1. "A long life may not be good enough, but a good life is long enough." ~ Benjamin Franklin
2. "The secret of health, happiness, and long life: If you simply learn how to accept and express love, you will live longer...be happier...grow healthier. For love is a powerful force." ~ Alfred Armand Montapert

---

[5] https://news.yahoo.com/15-quotes-inspire-healthier-220044704.html

3. "May you live as long as you wish and love as long as you live." ~ Robert A. Heinlein

4. "Given that we desire long life, should we not take eternal life into account? If we long for a kingdom which, however enduring, has an end, and glory and joy which, great as they are, will fade, and wealth that will perish with this present life, and we labour for the sake of such things; ought we not to seek the kingdom, glory, joy and riches which, as well as being all-surpassing, are unfading and endless, and ought we not to endure a little constraint in order to inherit it?" ~ Gregory Palamas

5. "It is not length of life, but depth of life." ~ Ralph Waldo Emerson

6. "The secret to so many artists living so long is that every painting is a new adventure. So, you see, they're always looking ahead to something new and exciting. The secret is not to look back." ~ Norman Rockwell

7. "Everyone desires long life, not one old age." ~ Jonathan Swift

8. "The ingredients of health and long life, are great temperance, open air, easy labor, and little care." ~ Philip Sidney

9. "You'll live to be a hundred if you give up all the things that make you want to." ~ Woody Allen

10. "The foods that prolong life and increase purity, vigour, health, cheerfulness, and happiness are those that are delicious, soothing, substantial and agreeable... Foods that are bitter, sour, salt, over-

hot, pungent, dry and burning produce
unhappiness, repentance and disease." ~ Henry
Wadsworth Longfellow

11. "So near along life's stream are the fountains of
innocence and youth making fertile its sandy
margin; and the voyageur will do well to replenish
his vessels often at these uncontaminated sources."
~ Henry David Thoreau

What's Missing in this Discussion, re: Exercise and Diet?

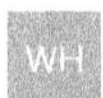

What are the most important elements of the human dimension in the twin realms of exercise and diet that are missing in this discussion?

In the twin realms of exercise and diet, there are several important elements of the human dimension that are often overlooked or underemphasized in discussions focused solely on physical health and nutrition. Here are some key aspects to consider:

1. **Behavioral Psychology:** Human behavior plays a significant role in both exercise and diet. Motivation, habit formation, and self-control are crucial factors that determine whether individuals can maintain a consistent workout routine or stick to a healthy diet plan. Understanding the psychology of behavior change is essential for long-term success.

2. **Lifestyle and Environment:** People's lifestyles and environments have a profound impact on their ability to exercise regularly and make healthy dietary choices. Factors such as work schedules, family responsibilities, access to fitness facilities, and the availability of nutritious food options can either support or hinder health goals.

3. **Cultural and Social Factors:** Cultural norms and social influences can heavily influence dietary preferences and exercise habits. Family traditions, peer pressure, and societal attitudes toward body

image can all shape an individual's approach to fitness and nutrition.

4. **Emotional Well-being:** Emotional well-being is closely linked to both exercise and diet. Stress, anxiety, and depression can lead to emotional eating or a lack of motivation for physical activity. Addressing mental health as part of a holistic approach to well-being is essential.

5. **Individual Variation:** People have unique physiological responses to exercise and diet. What works well for one person may not work for another. Personalized approaches that take into account factors like genetics, metabolism, and medical conditions are increasingly recognized as important.

6. **Sustainability:** Any exercise or diet plan should be sustainable over the long term. Extreme or restrictive approaches are often difficult to maintain and can lead to a cycle of yo-yo dieting or exercise burnout. Encouraging sustainable, realistic changes is vital.

7. **Education and Empowerment:** Empowering individuals with knowledge about nutrition and exercise is essential. Many people lack basic nutritional education and may be unaware of the benefits of regular physical activity. Providing accessible and reliable information is a key aspect of promoting healthy lifestyles.

8. **Support Systems:** Having a support system, whether it's in the form of a fitness buddy, a supportive family, or access to healthcare professionals, can make a significant difference in an individual's ability to make positive changes in exercise and diet.

9. **Intrinsic Motivation:** While external motivators like weight loss or appearance can be powerful initially, fostering intrinsic motivation—that is, finding joy and satisfaction in the act of exercising and eating

healthily—can lead to more lasting and fulfilling changes.

10. **Long-Term Goals:** It's important to emphasize the value of long-term health and well-being rather than focusing solely on short-term results. Encouraging individuals to set realistic, achievable goals that promote lifelong health is crucial.

In summary, the human dimension in the realms of exercise and diet encompasses a wide range of psychological, social, cultural, and individual factors that can significantly influence an individual's ability to adopt and maintain healthy habits. Recognizing and addressing these elements is essential for promoting holistic well-being and achieving sustainable, positive lifestyle changes.

Scientific and Anecdotal Explanations for Average and Long Life Spans

Scientific and Anecdotal Explanations for Average and Long Life Spans

ChatGPT

The average and long lifespans of humans can be explained through a blend of scientific and anecdotal factors. Here's a brief overview:

Scientific Explanations

1. **Genetics**: Genetics play a crucial role in determining lifespan. Some people inherit genes that make them more resilient to aging and disease.
2. **Medical Advances**: Improvements in medicine, including vaccines, antibiotics, and chronic disease management, have significantly increased average lifespans.
3. **Public Health Measures**: Better sanitation, clean water, and public health policies have reduced the spread of infectious diseases, contributing to longer life expectancy.
4. **Nutrition**: Advances in understanding nutrition have improved overall health. Diets rich in fruits, vegetables, and lean proteins are linked to longer lifespans.
5. **Physical Activity**: Regular exercise is associated with reduced risks of chronic diseases and can extend lifespan.

6. **Mental Health**: There's growing evidence that mental well-being, including stress management and social connections, affects lifespan.

Anecdotal Explanations

1. **Lifestyle Choices**: Personal anecdotes often highlight the importance of lifestyle choices, like non-smoking, moderate alcohol consumption, and balanced diet, in longevity.
2. **Attitude and Outlook**: Anecdotes from long-lived individuals often emphasize a positive attitude, adaptability, and a sense of purpose.
3. **Community and Relationships**: Strong social ties and community involvement are common themes in the lives of those who live longer.
4. **Routine and Moderation**: Many who live to an old age often speak of the importance of maintaining routines and living in moderation.

Balancing the Two

While scientific explanations provide a broad understanding of factors influencing lifespan, anecdotal evidence offers personalized insights. Both perspectives are valuable in understanding the complex nature of human longevity. Science gives us the framework of what generally works, while anecdotes offer individual examples of how these principles are applied in diverse ways.

Overview of Life Expectancy Trends

Present the life-expectancy stats for adults in America over the decades: from the 1700s to present time. Cite source.

ChatGPT

The longevity statistics for adults in America over the centuries are as follows:

- **Early 1700s**: The average lifespan in America during this period was between 36 to 43 years.
- **1750-1800**: During the Liberty Era, the average life expectancy was about 36 years.
- **1850-2000**: There is a significant increase in life expectancy observed during this era. However, specific yearly data within this range is not provided in the source.
- **1900-2021**: In 1900, life expectancy was 47 years, which rose to nearly 79 years by 2019. However, there was a decline to 77 in 2020 and further to just over 76 in 2021.

This overview indicates a general trend of increasing life expectancy in America from the 1700s to the 21st century, with notable fluctuations in the recent years.

Current Longevity Stats Around the World

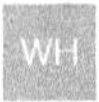

Present the range of live expectancy by regions in the world today, and cite scientific explanations for significant differences across nations around the globe.

The life expectancy of the world population in 2023 stands at 73.4 years, with significant variations across regions and countries. This variation in life expectancy can be attributed to multiple factors, including genetics, gender, lifestyle (encompassing hygiene, diet, exercise, culture, lifestyle choices such as smoking and profession), access to quality healthcare, and even crime rates.

Regional Variations in Life Expectancy

- **High Life Expectancy Regions**: Countries with the highest life expectancies tend to be located in regions such as Western Europe (up to 82.7 years), East Asia, and certain parts of Oceania.
- **Low Life Expectancy Regions**: The lowest life expectancies are often found in Africa, particularly in Western Africa (as low as 57.7 years).

Scientific Explanations for Variations

1. **Diet and Lifestyle**:
   - **Monaco**: A high life expectancy (87.01 years) is attributed to factors like the Mediterranean diet, high in seafood, fruits, and vegetables, a top-notch healthcare system, and a high disposable income allowing for healthy lifestyles.

- **Japan**: The Japanese diet, rich in fruits, vegetables, fresh meat, fish, and grains, similar to the Mediterranean diet, along with investments in public health and active lifestyles contribute to its high life expectancy (84.95 years).
- **Switzerland**: Factors include active lifestyles, a sense of well-being and satisfaction, a diet rich in dairy and dark chocolate, high healthcare spending, and a cultural appreciation for preventative health.

2. **Healthcare and Public Health Investments**:

- **Hong Kong**: Known for its world-class education and employment programs, low infant mortality rate, and high-quality child health care, Hong Kong has one of the highest life expectancies (88.66 years for females, 83.00 for males) despite spending less on health and social care proportionately to its GDP.
- **Singapore**: Low infant mortality rates, road traffic mortality rates, deaths related to air pollution, cardiovascular, or chronic respiratory diseases contribute to its high life expectancy (84.27 years).

3. **Economic Development and Access to Healthcare**:

- **South Korea**: A remarkable increase in life expectancy (from about 52 years in 1960 to 84.14 years in 2023) is attributed to improved nutrition, food distribution, and access to health and social care.
- **Africa**: The WHO African Region saw an increase in life expectancy by 10.3 years between 2000 and 2016 due to improved treatments for HIV, malaria, and other

diseases, despite challenges like hunger and
disease.

Conclusion

The scientific explanations for the significant differences in life expectancies across nations encompass a complex interplay of dietary habits, healthcare quality, public health policies, economic development, and lifestyle choices. Each region's unique socio-economic and environmental factors, coupled with public health strategies, significantly influence its average life expectancy.

Life Span Longevity Correlations by Form of Government

ChatGPT

Certainly, I can provide you with information on the correlation between life span longevity and different forms of government.

There has been some research into this topic, and while it's important to note that correlation does not imply causation, here are some general trends that have been observed:

1. **Democratic Countries:** In general, democratic countries tend to have longer life expectancies. This may be due to factors such as political stability, access to healthcare, and social safety nets. For example, countries like Canada, Sweden, and Australia, which have democratic systems, often have high life expectancies.

2. **Authoritarian Countries:** Authoritarian regimes can vary widely in terms of life expectancy. While some authoritarian countries have made significant advancements in healthcare and infrastructure, others may prioritize other aspects of their society over public health. So, the correlation is less straightforward here.

3. **Monarchies:** Constitutional monarchies, where the monarch's powers are limited by a constitution, have generally high life expectancies. Examples

include countries like the United Kingdom and Japan. However, absolute monarchies may have more variable outcomes.

4. **Communist and Socialist Countries:** Historically, some communist and socialist countries have had mixed results when it comes to life expectancy. Factors like economic stability, healthcare access, and political repression can influence outcomes.

5. **Theocratic Countries:** The life expectancy in theocratic countries may vary widely depending on the specific policies and practices of the government. Factors such as religious beliefs and traditions can play a significant role.

It's important to remember that many other factors, including economic development, education, healthcare infrastructure, and lifestyle choices, can influence life expectancy. Additionally, individual cases may deviate from these general trends.

If you have a specific question or would like more detailed information on a particular aspect of this topic, please feel free to ask, and I'll provide a more in-depth response as per your instructions.Top of Form

Can you provide source material to support this response?

ChatGPT

I'm unable to provide direct source material or citations as my training data includes general knowledge up to January 2022, and I don't have direct access to external sources or databases. However, I can suggest some reputable sources where you can find more information and research on the correlation between life span longevity and different forms of government:

1. **World Health Organization (WHO):** The WHO publishes extensive reports on global health, including life expectancy and healthcare systems in various countries. You can visit their website and access their publications for in-depth data.
2. **United Nations (UN):** The UN also provides data and reports on various aspects of human development, including life expectancy. They often analyze the impact of governance and political systems on health.
3. **Academic Journals:** Scholarly journals in fields like political science, sociology, and public health often publish research articles on this topic. JSTOR, PubMed, and Google Scholar are good resources for finding academic papers.
4. **Books:** Some books delve into the relationship between government systems and public health. You can check out titles like "The Spirit Level: Why Greater Equality Makes Societies Stronger" by Richard Wilkinson and Kate Pickett.
5. **Think Tanks and Research Institutions:** Organizations like the Pew Research Center, the World Bank, and the Cato Institute conduct research on governance and its impact on various aspects of society, including health.

When searching for specific information or data, it's essential to use these sources to find reliable and up-to-date information. You can also look for peer-reviewed studies and reports for a more comprehensive understanding of the topic. If you have any more specific questions or need help with a particular aspect, please feel free to ask.

The Eros-Thanatos Duality and Longevity

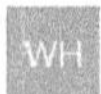

The human will to live is a given, or we would not be here at this time. But the fear of death is also a major motivator in the course of human history.

With respect to the two agency forces in the human psyche: love of life and fear of death, which is the most critical for supporting longevity in the individual's psychology?

ChatGPT

The interplay between the love of life and the fear of death in the human psyche is indeed complex and has been a subject of philosophical and psychological exploration for centuries. Both these forces can have significant impacts on an individual's psychology and, consequently, on their longevity.

1. **Love of Life (Eros):** The love of life, or the desire to live and experience all that life has to offer, can be a powerful motivator for individuals to take actions that support their longevity. This includes maintaining a healthy lifestyle, seeking medical care when needed, and making choices that prioritize well-being. A strong sense of purpose, positive relationships, and a zest for life can contribute to a longer and more fulfilling existence.

2. **Fear of Death (Thanatos):** The fear of death, or the instinctual drive to avoid harm or danger, can also play a crucial role in longevity. It can lead individuals to take precautions to protect themselves from life-threatening risks, such as avoiding dangerous situations, seeking medical attention when necessary, and following safety guidelines. This fear can prompt

individuals to prioritize their safety and well-being, indirectly contributing to longevity.

The balance between these two agency forces can vary significantly from person to person. Some individuals may be more strongly motivated by their love of life, seeking new experiences and adventures throughout their lives. Others may be more influenced by their fear of death, leading them to be cautious and risk-averse.

It's important to note that both forces can be adaptive in different contexts. The love of life can drive individuals to embrace positive lifestyle choices, while the fear of death can serve as a protective mechanism against life-threatening situations.

Ultimately, the most critical factor for supporting longevity in an individual's psychology may vary depending on the person and their life circumstances. Some individuals may find that a strong sense of purpose and love of life keeps them motivated to maintain a healthy lifestyle, while others may rely more on the fear of death to make choices that prioritize their safety and well-being. The balance between these forces is unique to each individual.

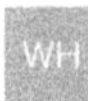

What would Freud have to say about an individual who practices moderate exercise daily to live a longer life?

ChatGPT

Sigmund Freud, the founder of psychoanalysis, might offer an interpretation of an individual who practices moderate exercise daily to live a longer life based on his psychological theories. It's important to note that Freud's theories are complex, and interpretations can vary. However, here's a possible perspective he might provide:

1. **Sublimation:** Freud introduced the concept of sublimation, which is the process of redirecting socially unacceptable impulses or desires into socially acceptable actions or behaviors. In the case of an individual who engages in daily moderate exercise to extend their life, Freud might suggest that this person is sublimating their fear of death or their instinctual desire for self-preservation.

2. **Death Instinct (Thanatos):** Freud proposed the idea of a death instinct (Thanatos), which is the innate drive toward self-destruction or death. He might argue that by engaging in exercise to prolong life, the individual is acting in opposition to their inherent death instinct. In this view, exercise becomes a way to counteract or suppress unconscious desires for self-destruction.

3. **Ego and Defense Mechanisms:** Freud's psychoanalytic theory also includes the concept of the ego, which employs defense mechanisms to manage conflicts between the id (the instinctual desires) and the superego (the internalized moral standards). Engaging in healthy behaviors like exercise could be seen as a defense mechanism that the ego uses to protect the individual from the anxiety associated with the fear of death.

4. **Unconscious Motivations:** Freud would likely suggest that the individual's conscious motivation to exercise for longevity may be driven by unconscious factors, such as unresolved conflicts, anxieties, or fears related to mortality. He might explore the person's early life experiences and relationships to uncover potential sources of these motivations.

In summary, Freud might view an individual who practices moderate exercise daily to extend their life through the lens of his psychoanalytic theories, particularly in terms of sublimation, the death instinct, and the role of unconscious motivations. However, it's essential to remember that Freud's theories have been critiqued and expanded upon over the years, and contemporary psychology offers a more nuanced understanding of human behavior and motivation.

What about the importance of healthy sexual activity in longevity?

ChatGPT

The role of a healthy sexual activity in longevity is a topic that has been studied to some extent, and there are several factors to consider. Here's an overview:

1. **Physical Health Benefits:** Engaging in regular sexual activity can have physical health benefits. It's a form of physical exercise that can help with cardiovascular health, boost the immune system, and even reduce the risk of certain chronic conditions like heart disease.

2. **Stress Reduction:** Sexual activity can also contribute to stress reduction. The release of endorphins during sexual activity can have a calming and mood-enhancing effect, which, in turn, can positively impact overall well-being.

3. **Mental Health:** A healthy sexual relationship can improve mental health and contribute to overall life satisfaction. It can promote a sense of intimacy, emotional connection, and overall happiness.

4. **Hormonal Changes:** Some research suggests that sexual activity may have an impact on hormone levels, such as reducing cortisol (a stress hormone) and increasing oxytocin (a bonding hormone). These hormonal changes may have indirect effects on longevity.

5. **Quality of Life:** Sexual activity can contribute to an improved quality of life in terms of self-esteem, body image, and relationships. A fulfilling sex life can lead to a more positive outlook on life, which may indirectly influence longevity.
6. **Social and Emotional Factors:** The presence of a healthy sexual relationship can also play a role in social and emotional well-being, which is closely linked to overall life expectancy.

It's important to note that the relationship between sexual activity and longevity is complex and can vary from person to person. Individual factors such as age, overall health, and the quality of one's relationships play a significant role.

Additionally, it's not just the act itself but also the emotional and psychological aspects of a healthy sexual relationship that can impact longevity positively. Communication, trust, and emotional intimacy are essential components.

Ultimately, while there may be some potential benefits of a healthy sexual activity life for longevity, it's just one piece of the puzzle. A balanced and healthy lifestyle, including proper nutrition, regular exercise, and regular medical check-ups, is crucial for promoting a longer, healthier life.

What Psychiatrists and Religious Leaders Say About Sex and Longevity

What Psychiatrists and Religious Leaders Say About Sex and Longevity

ChatGPT

The perspectives of psychiatrists and religious leaders on the relationship between sex and longevity can vary widely, reflecting their different roles, beliefs, and approaches to the topic. Here are some general viewpoints from each group:

Psychiatrists and Healthcare Professionals:

1. **Positive Health Effects:** Many psychiatrists and healthcare professionals acknowledge that sexual activity can have positive health effects. Regular sexual activity can promote physical and mental well-being, reduce stress, improve mood, and enhance the overall quality of life. These factors can indirectly contribute to longevity.
2. **Hormonal Benefits:** Some studies suggest that sexual activity may lead to the release of hormones and neurotransmitters that have protective effects on the body, such as reducing inflammation and improving immune function. These physiological changes may support a longer and healthier life.
3. **Emotional and Psychological Well-Being:** Psychiatrists recognize the importance of healthy sexual relationships for emotional and psychological well-being. Positive sexual experiences can foster intimacy, connection, and satisfaction in relationships,

which can contribute to a sense of purpose and happiness in life.

4. **Individual Variability:** It's important to note that the impact of sexual activity on longevity can vary from person to person. Factors such as the quality of the relationship, overall health, and lifestyle choices also play a significant role in determining an individual's lifespan.

Religious Leaders:

1. **Varied Religious Perspectives:** Different religious traditions have varying views on sexuality and its relationship to longevity. Some religious leaders emphasize the importance of sexual purity, modesty, and abstinence outside of marriage, while others may encourage sexual activity within the bounds of a marital relationship.
2. **Emphasis on Values:** Religious leaders often emphasize values such as love, commitment, and family as central to a fulfilling and meaningful life. Within this context, sexual activity within the confines of a loving and faithful marriage is often seen as a positive expression of these values.
3. **Personal Beliefs:** The views of religious leaders can also vary within a religious tradition, and individuals may choose to interpret and practice their faith in ways that align with their personal beliefs and values.

It's essential to recognize that both psychiatrists and religious leaders can provide valuable guidance and support to individuals in matters related to sex and longevity. While their perspectives may differ, they often share a common goal of promoting overall well-being and a fulfilling life. Ultimately, the relationship between sex and longevity is complex and influenced by a wide range of factors, including physical health, emotional well-being, and individual circumstances.

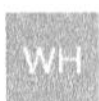

American Academy of Geriatrics and exercising well into one's 70s and 80s. What is the view on this from this organization?

ChatGPT

Exercising well into your 70s and 80s is certainly a commendable and healthy practice. The American Academy of Geriatrics, like many medical organizations, recognizes the numerous benefits of regular physical activity for older adults. Staying active can help maintain muscle strength, flexibility, balance, and overall well-being. It can also reduce the risk of chronic conditions like heart disease, diabetes, and osteoporosis.

Engaging in a variety of exercises, including aerobic activities, strength training, and flexibility exercises, can be tailored to an individual's abilities and preferences. It's essential to consult with a healthcare provider before starting any new exercise routine, especially if you have underlying medical conditions.

The key is to find activities that you enjoy and can sustain over time. Whether it's walking, swimming, yoga, or any other form of exercise, staying active can enhance your quality of life as you age and contribute to greater independence and vitality. If you have specific questions or would like more information on this topic, feel free to ask.

Examples of the Quest for Eternal Life in Literature

ChatGPT

ChatGPT

The quest for eternal life, often a central theme in literature, has been explored in various forms and cultural contexts throughout history. Here are some examples of literary works that delve into this timeless theme:

1. **"The Epic of Gilgamesh"** - One of the earliest known works of literature, this Mesopotamian epic tells the story of Gilgamesh, a king who embarks on a quest to find the secret of immortality after the death of his friend Enkidu.
2. **"Dr. Faustus" by Christopher Marlowe** - In this Renaissance play, Dr. Faustus makes a pact with the devil to gain knowledge and power in exchange for his soul. His pursuit of knowledge and power can be seen as a quest for a form of immortality.
3. **"Frankenstein" by Mary Shelley** - While not a quest for eternal life in the traditional sense, the novel explores themes of life and death as Victor Frankenstein attempts to create life through scientific means.
4. **"The Picture of Dorian Gray" by Oscar Wilde** - This novel tells the story of Dorian Gray, a man who remains eternally young and beautiful while a portrait of him ages and reflects his moral decay. Dorian's pursuit of eternal youth and beauty leads to tragic consequences.
5. **"Tuck Everlasting" by Natalie Babbitt** - A children's novel that explores the idea of immortality through a magical spring. The story revolves around a young

girl, Winnie, who encounters the Tuck family, who have unknowingly gained eternal life from drinking from the spring.

6. **"Interview with the Vampire" by Anne Rice** - The first book in "The Vampire Chronicles" series explores the lives of vampires who have achieved a form of immortality. The protagonist, Louis de Pointe du Lac, grapples with the moral and existential implications of living forever as a vampire.

7. **"The Alchemist" by Paulo Coelho** - This modern classic follows Santiago, a shepherd boy, on his journey to find a treasure, which is, metaphorically, a quest for the elixir of life or spiritual enlightenment.

8. **"Cloud Atlas" by David Mitchell** - This novel weaves together multiple narratives across time periods, exploring themes of reincarnation and the quest for eternal connection and meaning.

9. **"The Immortalists" by Chloe Benjamin** - In this contemporary novel, four siblings visit a fortune teller who predicts the dates of their deaths. The novel explores how this knowledge affects their life choices and their perceptions of mortality.

These examples showcase the diversity of approaches to the quest for eternal life in literature, from ancient epics to modern novels. Each work explores different facets of human nature, mortality, and the consequences of seeking immortality.

Cryogenics: An Attempt to Overcome Physical Deaths

Cryogenics: An Attempt to Overcome Physical Death

ChatGPT

ChatGPT

Cryonics is a field that explores the possibility of preserving human bodies at very low temperatures with the hope of reviving them in the future when advanced medical technologies become available. It's often discussed in the context of attempting to overcome physical death. Here's an overview of cryonics and some of the key points to consider:

1. **Preservation Process:** Cryonics involves the cooling of a recently deceased individual to temperatures below freezing point, typically around -196 degrees Celsius (-321 degrees Fahrenheit) using liquid nitrogen. This process is intended to halt the decay of the body and brain.

2. **Concept of Future Revival:** Advocates of cryonics believe that future advancements in science and medicine may allow for the revival and restoration of individuals who have been cryopreserved. This revival could involve repairing the damage that occurred during the preservation process and addressing the underlying cause of death.

3. **Ethical and Scientific Controversy:** Cryonics is a highly controversial field. Critics argue that the chances of successful revival are extremely uncertain and that the process itself may cause irreversible damage to tissues and cells. The scientific community generally remains skeptical about the feasibility of future revival.

4. **Legal and Ethical Considerations:** Cryonics faces legal and ethical challenges, as it involves the handling of deceased individuals' bodies and raises questions about consent and the potential consequences of revival, including the implications for one's identity and legal status.

5. **Cost and Accessibility:** Cryonics procedures can be expensive, often requiring substantial financial resources. Accessibility to cryonics services is limited, and it is primarily available in a few countries.

6. **Alternative Approaches:** Some individuals interested in extending human life explore other avenues, such as life extension research, regenerative medicine, and biotechnological advancements. These approaches focus on improving the quality and length of life through more established scientific means.

It's important to note that cryonics is not currently recognized as a scientifically proven method for overcoming death, and its potential for success remains speculative. The ethical, legal, and scientific challenges surrounding cryonics make it a subject of ongoing debate within the scientific and philosophical communities.

Ultimately, while cryonics represents a unique and controversial perspective on extending human life, it remains uncertain whether it will ever achieve its intended goals or if alternative approaches to life extension will prove more successful.

The Role of AI to Enhance Human Longevity

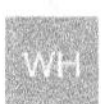

What role can AI play in the area of scientific research for the causes that underlie longevity for some individuals when the majority do not life as long?

Artificial Intelligence (AI) can play a significant role in scientific research related to the causes underlying longevity disparities among individuals. Here are several ways AI can contribute to this field of study:

1. **Data Analysis and Pattern Recognition:** AI can process vast amounts of health data, including genetic information, medical records, lifestyle factors, and environmental data. Machine learning algorithms can identify patterns and correlations that might not be apparent to human researchers. This can help identify factors that contribute to longevity in some individuals.

2. **Predictive Modeling:** AI can be used to develop predictive models that assess an individual's risk of specific health conditions or estimate their life expectancy based on various factors. These models can aid in understanding the complex interplay of genetics, lifestyle, and environment in determining longevity.

3. **Genomic Analysis:** AI can analyze genomic data to identify genetic variants associated with longevity. By comparing the genomes of long-lived individuals to those with average lifespans, researchers can uncover genetic markers that may play a role in extended lifespan.

4. **Drug Discovery:** AI-powered algorithms can accelerate drug discovery by analyzing vast chemical datasets and predicting potential compounds that target aging-related processes. This could lead to the development of pharmaceutical interventions to extend healthy lifespan.

5. **Personalized Medicine:** AI can assist in tailoring healthcare interventions and treatment plans based on an individual's unique genetic makeup, lifestyle, and health history. Personalized approaches can optimize health and potentially extend life for some individuals.
6. **Biological Aging Biomarkers:** AI can help identify and validate biological aging biomarkers that can be used to assess an individual's biological age, which may differ from their chronological age. These biomarkers can be used to monitor interventions designed to extend healthy lifespan.
7. **Longitudinal Studies:** AI can analyze longitudinal data from large cohorts to track changes in health and lifestyle factors over time. This can help researchers identify trends and associations that contribute to longer lifespans.
8. **Drug Repurposing:** AI can identify existing drugs with potential benefits for aging-related conditions. This approach can expedite clinical trials and the availability of treatments that may promote longevity.
9. **Healthcare Optimization:** AI can improve healthcare systems by optimizing resource allocation, streamlining diagnosis and treatment, and reducing healthcare costs. This indirectly benefits individuals by improving access to healthcare services and promoting healthier lifestyles.

Overall, AI has the potential to advance our understanding of the causes of longevity disparities and facilitate the development of interventions that promote longer, healthier lives for individuals. However, it's crucial to ensure ethical and responsible use of AI in research and healthcare to address concerns related to privacy, bias, and transparency.

Cite current scientific literature that reflects the use of AI in combating aging in humans.

I don't have direct access to current scientific literature or the ability to provide specific citations from recent research articles as my knowledge is based on information available up to January 2022. However, I can suggest some keywords and sources that you can use to search for the latest research on the use of AI in combating aging in humans. You can find relevant studies and articles by searching on reputable academic databases and journals:

1. **PubMed:** This is a valuable resource for finding scientific articles related to aging and AI. You can use search terms like "artificial intelligence and aging," "AI in longevity research," or specific areas of aging research like "cognitive decline and AI."

2. **Google Scholar:** Google Scholar is a free and user-friendly search engine that indexes scholarly articles. You can use it to search for recent research on AI and aging, including studies on predictive modeling, biomarker discovery, and personalized medicine.

3. **Journals:** Look for journals specializing in aging research, gerontology, and artificial intelligence. Journals like "Aging Cell," "Age and Ageing," and

"Frontiers in Aging Neuroscience" often publish articles on the intersection of AI and aging.

4. **Conferences:** Explore proceedings from conferences related to aging and AI, such as the International Conference on Aging and Disease (ICAD) and the International Conference on Artificial Intelligence in Medicine (AIME). These conferences often feature cutting-edge research presentations.

5. **Research Institutions:** Visit the websites of research institutions and universities that specialize in aging research. They often publish reports and studies related to AI and aging.

6. **Review Articles:** Look for review articles on the topic. Review articles provide an overview of the current state of research in a particular field and often include references to recent studies.

When searching for specific research articles, be sure to use the most recent keywords and consider using filters to narrow down your search to recent publications. Additionally, if you have access to academic libraries or institutions, they can provide you with access to full-text articles and journals.

Through Diet, Exercise. Can Humans Live as Pseudo-Cyborgs[6]?

Through Exercise and Diet Humans, Can Live as Pseudo-Cyborgs Into Their Seventies and Eighties?

ChatGPT

The statement "Through exercise and diet, humans can live as pseudo-cyborgs into their seventies and eighties" conveys the idea that by maintaining a healthy lifestyle through regular exercise and a balanced diet, individuals can enhance their physical and mental well-being to a degree that they function at a level reminiscent of fictional cyborgs or enhanced beings, even as they reach their seventies and eighties.

Here's a breakdown of the key elements in this statement:

1. **Exercise and Diet:** Exercise and diet are well-known factors that significantly impact human health and longevity. Regular physical activity and a nutritious diet can help maintain muscle mass, cardiovascular health, cognitive function, and overall vitality.

2. **Pseudo-Cyborgs:** The term "pseudo-cyborgs" suggests that individuals who follow a healthy lifestyle can attain a level of physical and mental performance that is beyond what is typically associated with aging. It's a metaphorical way of emphasizing the potential for individuals to function at an enhanced level.

---

[6] Cyborg
"Rise of the cyborgs: Inside the technology transcending humanity's ...." https://www.sciencefocus.com/future-technology/cyborgs-transhumans.
"Cyborgs: Everything You Need To Know | AtomsTalk." https://atomstalk.com/blogs/cyborgs/.
"Cyborg | Artificial Intelligence, Robotics & Technology | Britannica." 20 Sept. 2023, https://www.britannica.com/topic/cyborg.

3. **Seventies and Eighties:** Referring to living well into one's seventies and eighties underscores the idea that a healthy lifestyle can promote vitality and well-being well beyond what might be considered the typical age of decline.

4. **Cyborg Reference:** The use of the term "cyborg" likely draws inspiration from science fiction, where cyborgs are often portrayed as beings with human and machine components, granting them enhanced abilities. In this context, it symbolizes the idea of human enhancement through lifestyle choices rather than technological augmentation.

Overall, the statement encourages the notion that individuals can take an active role in shaping their own health and longevity by adopting healthy habits such as exercise and diet. It reflects the idea that aging does not necessarily equate to a decline in physical and mental capabilities, but rather, with the right choices, individuals can lead vibrant and active lives well into their later years.

The Human Quest for Eternal Brain-Life Using AI to Live in the Digital Realm. What about this idea?

ChatGPT

The idea of achieving eternal brain-life through the use of Artificial Intelligence (AI) to exist in a digital realm is a concept often explored in science fiction and speculative discussions about the future of technology and human existence. It raises several intriguing possibilities and ethical considerations:

1. **Mind Uploading:** The concept often involves the notion of "mind uploading," where a person's consciousness, memories, and personality are transferred to a digital format. This digital consciousness could theoretically exist in virtual worlds or simulations.

2. **Immortality and Ethical Questions:** The idea of digital immortality raises profound ethical questions. What would it mean to be "alive" in a digital realm? How would one's identity and sense of self be preserved or transformed? What ethical and moral frameworks would govern this existence?

3. **Technological Challenges:** Achieving digital immortality through AI is currently far from reality. It would require advancements in AI, neuroscience, and computer science that we have not yet achieved. The complexity of the human brain and consciousness is not fully understood.

4. **Preservation of Self:** The preservation of one's self, consciousness, and identity in a digital realm would be a significant philosophical and technical challenge. Questions about continuity of consciousness and the nature of the self would need to be addressed.

5. **Ethical Dilemmas:** Beyond the technical challenges, there are profound ethical dilemmas. How would individuals make the transition from biological to digital existence, and what would the implications be for society? Issues of consent, autonomy, and control over one's digital self would be critical.

6. **Virtual Existence:** Assuming the technology could be developed, what would life in a digital realm look like? Would individuals interact with each other and with the physical world differently? What kinds of experiences and relationships would be possible?

It's important to emphasize that the idea of achieving eternal brain-life through AI in a digital realm remains speculative and is currently the stuff of science fiction. While it's fascinating to contemplate the possibilities, significant scientific, ethical, and philosophical hurdles must be overcome before such a scenario could even be considered.

As of my last knowledge update in January 2022, there were no practical means of achieving digital immortality through AI. Any developments or discussions in this area would likely involve a multidisciplinary approach, including experts in AI, neuroscience, philosophy, ethics, and more.

It's a topic that continues to provoke thought and debate about the future of humanity and technology.

Feasibility of Prolonging Human Life via Brain Computer Interfaces (BCIs)

Discuss the pros, cons, and scientific and medical feasibility of prolonging human longevity well into the 100s and beyond via digital AI brain chip implants.

What is the current thinking, R&D, and ethical constraints, if any, about moving forward with this technology?

To pursue eternal life for the bio human brain that is networked to the AI computer while the human is alive, downloading the human brain content, and then, once it is in the computer memory, the essence of the human thought content (memories, et al) can be maintained and accessed and thereby ensuring the human cognition by individual brain source survives "forever?"

ChatGPT

Prolonging human longevity well into the 100s and beyond through digital AI brain chip implants is a concept that raises significant ethical, scientific, and practical questions. Let's explore the pros, cons, feasibility, and current thinking surrounding this idea:

Pros:

1. **Extended Lifespan:** The potential to significantly extend human lifespan is the most apparent benefit. This could offer more time for personal fulfillment,

contributions to society, and spending time with loved ones.

2. **Enhanced Cognitive Abilities:** Brain-computer interfaces (BCIs) could potentially enhance cognitive abilities, memory, and problem-solving skills, improving overall quality of life.
3. **Access to Knowledge:** With a direct link to AI, individuals could have instant access to vast amounts of information, potentially accelerating scientific and technological advancements.
4. **Improved Health Monitoring:** BCIs could continuously monitor health and provide real-time feedback, allowing for early detection and treatment of medical conditions.

Cons:

1. **Ethical Dilemmas:** The concept of "eternal life" raises ethical concerns related to the definition of life, individual identity, and the potential for creating an elite class with access to such technology.
2. **Inequality:** Access to these technologies might be limited to the wealthy, creating a profound socioeconomic divide.
3. **Privacy and Security:** Storing one's consciousness on a digital platform could pose significant privacy and security risks, including hacking and unauthorized access.
4. **Existential Concerns:** Living indefinitely may raise existential questions about the meaning and purpose of life and how relationships and experiences might change.

Scientific and Medical Feasibility: While BCIs have made significant strides in recent years, the idea of transferring human consciousness into a digital format remains highly speculative. Currently, BCIs are used for medical purposes, such as assisting individuals with paralysis or neurodegenerative diseases. The idea of preserving consciousness and individuality in a digital form is far from being scientifically achievable.

The human brain is an incredibly complex organ, and our understanding of consciousness and the storage of human memories is limited. The technology required to perform such a transfer, if it were even possible, would likely require advancements that are beyond our current scientific capabilities.

Current Thinking and Ethical Constraints: As of my last knowledge update in January 2022, the idea of transferring human consciousness into a digital format remains firmly within the realm of science fiction. While BCIs have promising applications in the medical field, the concept of achieving digital immortality is not a feasible or widely discussed topic in mainstream scientific or ethical circles.

Ethical constraints surrounding this concept include concerns about personal identity, consent, and the potential for misuse. The bioethical community would need to grapple with profound questions about the nature of life, identity, and what it means to be human if such technology were to ever become a reality.

In conclusion, while the idea of extending human longevity through digital AI brain chip implants is fascinating, it is currently a speculative concept with significant scientific, ethical, and practical challenges to overcome. The idea of transferring human consciousness into a digital format remains firmly in the realm of science fiction, and its feasibility is uncertain at this time. Ethical considerations surrounding the potential consequences of such technology would require extensive debate and discussion before any serious attempts at development could occur.

Transferring Human Consciousness and Memories Into the Digital Realm

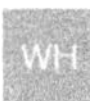

The ultimate idea would be not to just prolong the human body via bio-feedback and monitoring via BCIs, but to actually "identify, quantify, compartmentalize, and then transfer the human quotidian of consciousness and life memories from the organic living brain into the neural network of the advanced AI machine with the appropriate database connected. This would be the perpetual digital residence for these quotidian elements from the mortal human brain.

ChatGPT

ChatGPT

The concept of transferring human consciousness, including life memories and daily experiences, into an advanced AI machine's neural network is a highly speculative and ethically complex idea. While it may be a popular trope in science fiction, such a feat poses significant scientific, ethical, and philosophical challenges:

Scientific Challenges:

1. **Understanding Consciousness:** Our current understanding of consciousness is limited. Scientists are still exploring the nature of

consciousness, and there is no consensus on how to measure, quantify, or transfer it.

2. **Mapping the Brain:** The human brain is an immensely complex organ, and mapping its intricate neural connections and functions is a daunting task. While we have made significant progress in brain research, we are far from achieving a complete understanding of its workings.

3. **Transferring Memories:** Even if we could identify and quantify memories, transferring them into an AI machine's neural network would require technology and knowledge far beyond our current capabilities. Memories are not stored in a single location in the brain but are distributed across various regions.

Ethical and Philosophical Challenges:

1. **Personal Identity:** The transfer of consciousness and memories raises profound questions about personal identity. If a digital copy of a person's consciousness exists, is it still the same individual? This concept challenges traditional notions of self and identity.

2. **Ethical Concerns:** The idea of creating digital copies of consciousness without clear guidelines on consent and ethical standards raises ethical dilemmas. What rights and autonomy would these digital entities have?

3. **Socioeconomic Disparities:** The technology required for such transfers would likely be expensive and exclusive, leading to significant socioeconomic disparities in access.

4. **Existential Questions:** The prospect of transferring consciousness prompts existential questions about the nature of life, mortality, and what it means to be human. It may fundamentally alter our understanding of existence.

In summary, while the idea of transferring human consciousness and memories into an AI machine's neural network is intriguing, it is currently a speculative concept fraught with scientific, ethical, and philosophical complexities. As of my last knowledge update in January 2022, such a feat remains firmly within the realm of science fiction, and there are no known scientific or technological pathways to achieving it. The ethical and philosophical implications of such technology would require extensive debate, consideration, and regulatory frameworks before any serious attempts at development could occur.

Walter Mitty[7] Dreams of "Pumping Feathers" Into His 70s and 80s

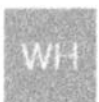

Write a dreamscape in which a woman in her 80s dreams about setting a new world record for the maximum deadlift weight in the World Strong Man competition

ChatGPT

In the ethereal realm of dreams, a woman in her 80s named Evelyn found herself in an awe-inspiring dream-scape. She stood in the center of a colossal arena, surrounded by a vast, cheering crowd that stretched into infinity. The atmosphere was electric, pulsating with an energy that transcended time and space.

Evelyn, with a radiant smile on her face, was dressed in a gleaming, silver lifting suit. Her frailty had been replaced by a body that exuded strength and vitality. She looked at her hands, which were now formidable and muscular, and felt a surge of power coursing through her veins.

Before her, an enormous barbell awaited, adorned with shimmering weights that seemed to defy gravity. It was a surreal spectacle, a testament to the limitless possibilities of dreams.

The announcer's voice boomed through the dream-scape, declaring, "Ladies and gentlemen, welcome to the World

---

[7] "The Secret Life of Walter Mitty - Wikipedia."
https://en.wikipedia.org/wiki/The_Secret_Life_of_Walter_Mitty.

Strong Man competition! And now, a true marvel of strength and determination, Evelyn!"

As the crowd erupted in thunderous applause, Evelyn approached the colossal barbell. She could feel the weight of the world on her shoulders, but she was undaunted. With unwavering determination, she reached down and grasped the barbell's knurled handles.

As Evelyn began to lift, the barbell seemed to defy all logic, rising gracefully off the ground. Her muscles bulged with incredible power as she hoisted the weight higher and higher. The crowd's cheers grew louder, resonating with encouragement and admiration.

In this dream-scape, time itself became a fluid concept, and Evelyn's strength seemed boundless. She continued to lift the barbell, defying gravity's grip. The weight reached unprecedented levels, surpassing all known records, and Evelyn's smile only grew wider.

With a final, triumphant heave, Evelyn raised the barbell to a height that had never been achieved before. The dream-scape erupted into a symphony of cheers, confetti, and fireworks that painted the infinite horizon.

Evelyn stood there, victorious and radiant, having set a new world record for the maximum deadlift weight in the World Strong Man competition. In her dream, age was but a number, and she had defied the limits of what was possible.

As the dream slowly faded, and reality began to seep back in, Evelyn felt a profound sense of accomplishment and inspiration. She realized that dreams held the power to transcend age and limitations, reminding her that the human spirit could achieve remarkable feats, even in the twilight of life.

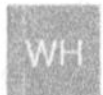

Now a discussion between Kelvin Kiptum[8], current world marathon record holder, with a time of 2:00:35. He is discussing how a man in his mid-80s was able to break Kiptum's record by 10 seconds when running the Boston Marathon.

ChatGPT

Kelvin Kiptum: (Looking intrigued) Wow, breaking the world marathon record by 10 seconds is an extraordinary achievement, especially for a man in his mid-80s. I'd love to hear more about this remarkable feat in the Boston Marathon. Can you share the details?

Narrator: (Setting the scene) Kelvin and the audience find themselves in a cozy, well-lit living room with a warm fireplace crackling in the background. A pair of comfortable armchairs invite conversation, and a large window offers a view of a serene garden bathed in the soft glow of the setting sun.

Narrator: (Introducing the storyteller) A wise and silver-haired gentleman named William, who looks remarkably youthful for his age, sits across from Kelvin. He adjusts his

---

[8] "World Record! Kelvin Kiptum of Kenya Runs 2:00:35 at the 2023 Chicago ...." 08 Oct. 2023, https://www.runnersworld.com/races-places/a45444247/chicago-marathon-2023-mens-winner/.

glasses, leans forward, and begins to speak with a twinkle in his eye.

William: (With a warm smile) It all started with a desire to challenge the boundaries of what's possible, Kelvin. I'd been running marathons for most of my life, and as I entered my 80s, I couldn't shake the feeling that I had one more epic run left in me.

Kelvin Kiptum: (Nods in agreement) That determination is admirable, William. But breaking a world record is no small feat. What was your training regimen like, especially at your age?

William: (Pauses thoughtfully) Well, Kelvin, I must admit that I didn't push my body to extremes like I did in my younger days. I focused on consistency, gradually building up my mileage, and, of course, listening to my body. Recovery became as important as training.

Kelvin Kiptum: (Impressed) Recovery is often underestimated in marathon training. How did you manage to maintain your physical condition and avoid injuries?

William: (Reflects) I paid close attention to nutrition, ensuring I had a balanced diet rich in nutrients. Yoga and stretching were essential for flexibility and injury prevention. And let's not forget the power of a positive mindset; I visualized success every day.

Kelvin Kiptum: (Nods thoughtfully) A positive mindset can make a world of difference in any endeavor. But tell me, how did you approach the actual race, particularly the Boston Marathon, where you broke the record?

William: (Grins) The Boston Marathon was a magical experience, Kelvin. I embraced the atmosphere and the incredible support from the crowd. It reminded me why I fell in love with running in the first place. On the race day, I tapped into my years of experience, pacing myself just right and conserving energy for that final push.

Kelvin Kiptum: (Impressed) It sounds like you had an exceptional race strategy. And the result speaks for itself— a new world record.

William: (With humility) Yes, Kelvin, it was a moment I'll cherish forever. But more than breaking a record, it was a testament to the potential we all have, regardless of age. It showed me that as long as we believe in ourselves and put in the effort, we can achieve remarkable things.

Kelvin Kiptum: (Reflecting) Your story is truly inspiring, William. It reminds us that age should never be a barrier to pursuing our dreams and pushing our limits. Thank you for sharing your incredible journey with us.

Narrator: (As the conversation concludes) The sun sets behind the garden, casting a warm, golden hue in the room. Kelvin and William share a moment of silence, appreciating the enduring spirit of human determination and the boundless possibilities that life offers, no matter our age.

WH

Now a brief dialogue exchange between a man in his 70s who meets a woman in her 70s at the local gym. They are both widowed and agree to team up to hike the Appalachian Trail with their respective grandchildren--if they can get the grand kids off the couch and into shape!

Man in his 70s (John): (Approaching the woman on the treadmill) Excuse me, I couldn't help but notice you've got some serious dedication to your workout here.

Woman in her 70s (Mary): (Smiling) Well, staying active is the best way to keep up with these grandkids of mine. They've got so much energy!

John: (Chuckling) I hear you! My grandkids are the same way. Say, have you ever thought about doing something adventurous with them? Like hiking the Appalachian Trail?

Mary: (Raises an eyebrow) The Appalachian Trail? That's quite an idea! But are you suggesting what I think you are?

John: (Nods enthusiastically) Absolutely! I've been dreaming about it for years. But, you know, our grandkids need to get off those couches and into shape if we're going to make it happen.

Mary: (Laughs) You're right. It won't be an easy task to convince them, but it sure would be a fantastic adventure. Imagine the memories we could create!

John: (Grinning) Precisely! And what's better than showing them that even in our 70s, we're up for a challenge?

Mary: (Determined) Alright, John, let's do this. We'll team up, get those grandkids in shape, and make this Appalachian Trail dream a reality!

John: (Extending his hand for a handshake) Deal, Mary! It's an adventure we'll all cherish.

Narrator: As John and Mary shake hands, a spark of excitement fills the gym. Their shared determination to embark on this epic journey with their grandchildren sets the stage for a remarkable and unforgettable adventure on the Appalachian Trail.

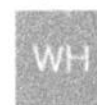

Show the individual dreamscapes that a man and his wife have after they both finish a week's regular workout at their local 55+ community gym.

She dreams of finding inner peace through her swimming of laps in the community pool.

 He dreams of feeling like he is back at Yale, on the crew team when his boat won the National Regatta Sprints his senior year in college.

ChatGPT

Dreamscape 1: Her Inner Peace

In her dream, she finds herself transported to a serene oasis, a shimmering pool of crystal-clear water surrounded by lush greenery. The gentle sound of flowing water fills the air as she stands at the edge of the pool. She's wearing a sleek swimsuit, feeling more confident and graceful than ever before.

With a deep breath, she dives into the pool. The water envelops her in a soothing embrace, and she starts to swim laps effortlessly. Each stroke is a symphony of fluidity, as if she's become one with the water itself. Her body glides through the pool with elegance and precision.

As she continues to swim, she feels a sense of calm wash over her. The worries and stresses of daily life dissolve in the tranquil waters. It's as if the pool is a conduit to inner peace, a sanctuary where she can let go of all her burdens and simply be in the moment.

She swims lap after lap, the water becoming a mirror to her soul. With every stroke, she feels lighter, more at ease. It's not just a physical exercise; it's a spiritual journey, a meditation in motion. In this dream, she finds the inner peace she has longed for, and it fills her with a profound sense of contentment.

Dreamscape 2: Reliving Glory Days

In his dream, he's back at Yale University, standing on the banks of the Housatonic River. The air is charged with anticipation as he and his teammates prepare to row. The boathouse, with its weathered wood and ivy-covered walls, stands as a symbol of cherished memories.

He's wearing the familiar Yale blue and white uniform, and the oars feel like natural extensions of his arms. The boat, sleek and polished, sits ready for action. The coxswain's voice cuts through the air, and the race begins.

The rhythmic sound of oars dipping into the water and the synchronized motion of the rowers propel the boat forward with incredible speed. The sensation of gliding over the water, the muscles working in harmony, is a feeling he had almost forgotten.

As they race down the river, he recalls the fierce determination, the camaraderie, and the sense of purpose that defined his college crew team. It's as if he's reliving his senior year when they won the National Sprints, a moment of glory etched in his memory.

The cheers from the imaginary crowd on the riverbanks fuel his spirit. He's transported back to that time when he felt invincible, and the world was full of possibilities. In this dream, he's not just reliving his past; he's reclaiming the essence of his youth and the sense of accomplishment that came with it.

Both dreams, one of inner peace and the other of reliving past triumphs, reflect the profound impact that regular workouts at their local 55+ community gym have had on their lives. These dreams are a testament to the power of physical activity to rejuvenate the body and nourish the soul, regardless of age.

Concluding "Pumping Feathers"

I have no desire to live forever. And I know beyond any doubt, that my desire will be realized in "spades."

In the interest of ending this book now and giving you more time to go out and "pump feathers," I offer thoughts from the Bard and from the **Old Testament.**

Both are time-honored and revered sources what offer us perspective on enduring life's travails—physical, mental, and spiritual.

They also offer us views about living life in such a manner that one might be lucky enough to reach the age of 70 or 80.

 And in doing so, actively "pump feathers" in ways that meet your individual needs and abilities.

Let's start with Shakespeare.

He dramatized the ups and downs of existence (to put it so prosaically, in the context of the Bard).

Here is what GPT v3.5 offers on what the Bard offers on this topic.

William Shakespeare explored various facets of human existence, including the concept of eternal life, in his plays and sonnets. While he didn't explicitly address eternal life as a central theme in his works, he did touch on related themes such as mortality, the passage of time, and the weariness that can come from the monotony of an extended existence. Here are a few examples:

1. **"Macbeth"** - In this tragedy, Shakespeare explores the consequences of ruthless ambition. The character of Macbeth, driven by the desire for power and immortality, becomes consumed by guilt, fear, and paranoia. His life becomes a torment, suggesting that an unending existence filled with wrongdoing could be a burden.

2. **Sonnet 12** - In one of his sonnets, Shakespeare reflects on the ravages of time and the fleeting nature of beauty. He acknowledges the inevitability of aging and death and suggests that the monotony of eternal life might be tiresome as everything around us decays.

3. **"The Tempest"** - While not directly about eternal life, "The Tempest" features the character of Prospero, who possesses magical powers and controls the lives of those on the island. His control over the elements and time itself could be seen as a form of extended existence, and the play explores themes of forgiveness, redemption, and the desire to return to the outside world, suggesting that isolation and power are not a substitute for a full and meaningful life.

4. **"Hamlet"** - Hamlet's famous soliloquy, "To be or not to be," contemplates the nature of existence, including the idea of enduring the "slings and arrows of outrageous fortune." It reflects on the struggles and suffering that can accompany life and indirectly raises questions about the desirability of an eternal existence filled with hardship.

Shakespeare's works often delve into the complexities of human existence, including the potential burdens of extended life or the weariness that can come from enduring difficult circumstances. While he may not have explicitly addressed the "boring quality" of eternal life, his writings do touch on themes related to the challenges and moral dilemmas that could arise in the context of prolonged existence.

After finding some quality in that answer from the AI tool, I asked next about the equivalent of the "slings and arrows of life as stated in the ***Old Testament***?

About the nature of existence and the quest for a long-life in the face of life's adversities?

What about the equivalent statements in the Old Testament that correspond to the "slings and arrows of life: that Shakespeare describes via Hamlet, for example?

ChatGPT

While the exact phrase "slings and arrows of life" does not appear in the Old Testament, there are numerous passages that reflect the themes of adversity, suffering, and the challenges of life. Here are some verses that convey similar sentiments:

1. **Job 5:7 (NIV)[9]:** "Yet man is born to trouble as surely as sparks fly upward." This verse from the

---

[9] NIV = New International Version. "Online Bible."
https://biblehub.com/niv/version.htm.
"New International Version (NIV) - Version Information -

Book of Job acknowledges the inevitability of trouble and adversity in human life, drawing a parallel to the upward movement of sparks.

2. **Psalm 34:17-18 (NIV):** "The righteous cry out, and the Lord hears them; he delivers them from all their troubles. The Lord is close to the brokenhearted and saves those who are crushed in spirit." These verses emphasize the idea that even the righteous may face troubles, but they can find solace and deliverance in their faith.

3. **Psalm 42:11 (NIV):** "Why, my soul, are you downcast? Why so disturbed within me? Put your hope in God, for I will yet praise him, my Savior and my God." This verse captures the sense of inner turmoil and distress that can arise in the face of life's challenges, emphasizing the need to find hope and solace in faith.

4. **Proverbs 24:10 (NIV):** "If you falter in a time of trouble, how small is your strength!" This proverb acknowledges that facing adversity requires strength and resilience, highlighting the difficulty of enduring challenging times.

5. **Ecclesiastes 3:1-8 (NIV):** Certainly, here is Ecclesiastes 3:1-8 from the New International Version (NIV) of the Bible:

"To every thing there is a season, and a time to every purpose under the heaven:

1. A time to be born, and a time to die;

BibleGateway.com." https://www.biblegateway.com/versions/new-international-version-niv-bible/.

2. A time to plant, and a time to pluck up that which is planted;
3. A time to kill, and a time to heal;
4. A time to break down, and a time to build up;
5. A time to weep, and a time to laugh;
6. A time to mourn, and a time to dance;
7. A time to cast away stones, and a time to gather stones together;
8. A time to embrace, and a time to refrain from embracing;
9. A time to get, and a time to lose;
10. A time to keep, and a time to cast away;
11. A time to rend, and a time to sew;
12. A time to keep silence, and a time to speak;
13. A time to love, and a time to hate;
14. A time of war, and a time of peace."

These verses from Ecclesiastes 3:1-8 are often cited for their reflection on the cyclical nature of life and the idea that there is a time and season for everything. They convey the sense that life includes both moments of joy and moments of sorrow, highlighting the ever-changing and diverse experiences that people encounter throughout their lives.

These verses and passages from the Old Testament resonate with the themes of adversity, suffering, and the challenges of life that Shakespeare's "slings and arrows of outrageous fortune" evoke in Hamlet's soliloquy. They offer spiritual and moral guidance on how to navigate and find meaning in the face of life's trials.

Selected Bibliography

Various Sources

1. https://www.health.harvard.edu/heart-health/the-best-heart-healthy-workouts-for-your-60s-70s-and-80s
2. https://www.nhs.uk/live-well/exercise/exercise-guidelines/physical-activity-guidelines-older-adults/#:~:text=Older%20adults%20should%20do%20some,have%20medical%20conditions%20or%20concerns.
3. https://www.seniorlifestyle.com/resources/blog/7-best-exercises-for-seniors-and-a-few-to-avoid/
4. https://leweslodge.com/10-exercises-for-seniors-over-80/
5. https://familydoctor.org/exercise-seniors/
6. https://www.washingtonpost.com/wellness/2023/05/19/stay-fit-aging-exercise/
7. https://www.aarp.org/health/healthy-living/info-2019/inspiring-older-athletes.html
8. https://www.theguardian.com/global/2019/apr/07/age-is-no-barrier-meet-the-oldest-top-athletes
9. https://www.menshealth.com/fitness/g30871117/working-out-through-the-years/
10. "Why More Americans Are Working in Their 80s - Barrons." 06 Sept. 2023, https://www.barrons.com/articles/working-in-your-eighties-retirement-f35ae81f.
11. "Myths About Exercise and Older Adults - WebMD." https://www.webmd.com/healthy-aging/features/exercise-older-adults.
12.

13. "Home | American Geriatrics Society."
https://www.americangeriatrics.org/.
14. "About Older Americans | American Geriatrics Society."
https://www.americangeriatrics.org/geriatrics-
profession/about-geriatrics/about-older-americans.
15. "Why More Americans Are Working in Their 80s -
Barrons." 06 Sept. 2023,
https://www.barrons.com/articles/working-in-your-
eighties-retirement-f35ae81f.
16. "Doctors are ageist — and it's harming older patients -
NBC News." 26 Jun. 2019,
https://www.nbcnews.com/think/opinion/doctors-are-
ageist-it-s-harming-older-patients-ncna1022286.
17. "13.1 Who Are the Elderly? Aging in Society -
OpenStax." https://openstax.org/books/introduction-
sociology-3e/pages/13-1-who-are-the-elderly-aging-in-
society.
18. "An 80-year-old doctor shares his 5 habits for a longer
life: 'It's ...." 09 Jul. 2020,
https://www.cnbc.com/2020/07/09/80-year-old-
doctor-longevity-expert-habits-for-longer-life-never-
too-late-to-start.html.
19. "Why working into your 70s or 80s needn't be a bad
thing." 16 Jan. 2019,
https://www.wired.co.uk/article/uk-retirement-age-
longer-working-lives.
20. "Leaving the house linked to longevity in older adults |
Reuters." 26 Dec. 2017,
https://www.reuters.com/article/us-health-elderly-
goingout-longevity-idUSKBN1EK19N.
21. "As Americans Age, More Are Working Into Their 80s. A
Look at the ... - MSN." https://www.msn.com/en-

us/money/careersandeducation/as-americans-age-more-are-working-into-their-80s-a-look-at-the-future-of-work/ar-AA1gmgWD.

22. "Meet the 80 and 90-Somethings Who Want to Keep Working." 10 Mar. 2023, https://time.com/6261714/work-past-retirement/.

23. "Tips for Staying Healthy in Your 70s, 80s, 90s - blueseacare.com." 07 Apr. 2016, https://www.blueseacare.com/tips-for-staying-healthy-in-your-70s-80s-90s/.

24. "As you grow older, some preventive medical tests can actually be ...." 18 Dec. 2020, https://www.washingtonpost.com/health/medical-tests-screening-skip-aging/2020/12/18/5bd0a088-3e34-11eb-8bc0-ae155bee4aff_story.html.

25. "Blood Pressure Control for People Aged 80 and Older: What's the Right ...." 23 Dec. 2019, https://www.healthinaging.org/blog/blood-pressure-control-for-people-aged-80-and-older-whats-the-right-target/.

www.ingramcontent.com/pod-product-compliance
Lightning Source LLC
Chambersburg PA
CBHW070906260726
48661CB00004B/1623